I0410453

Whole

Essentials

-Five Key Essentials to Change your Life-

Whole Essentials

Five Key Essentials to Change Your Life

Copyright © 2016 by Tiffnee Wertenberger

All rights reserved. No part of this book may be reproduced in any form or by any electronic or mechanical means, including information storage and retrieval systems, without permission in writing from the author. Headshot captured by Tallie Johnson Photography.

For information, contact Tiffnee Wertenberger at
tiffneewertenberger@gmail.com

The content of this book is for general informational purposes only. It is not meant to be used, nor should it be used, to diagnose or treat any medical condition or to replace the services of you physician or other health care providers. The advice and strategies contained in the book may not be suitable for all readers. Please consult your health care provider for any questions that you may have about your own medical situation. Neither the author, publisher, Institute for Integrative Nutrition nor any of their employees or representatives guarantees the accuracy of information in this book or its usefulness to a particular reader, nor are they responsible for any damages or negative consequences that may result from any treatment, action taken, or inaction by any person reading or following the information in this book.

ISBN- 13:978-1540345424

ISBN- 10:1540345424

Printed in the United States of America

Dedications

I dedicate this book to my wonderful parents. Their words of wisdom and love have guided me to where I am today.

From the bottom of my heart, thank you.

CONTENTS

Introduction

My health journey initially started when a doctor recommended a life-altering procedure! Dramatic? Yes, I know, yet what led to this visit was a series of not so dramatic events. Let me explain. I had a very normal and very happy childhood. I was blessed with amazing parents and a younger brother. We all ate three square American meals a day, got outside to play and always replenished with "sports drinks" as much as we did water. My brother and I played sports all year long, even raised farms animals and participated in 4H. We got cavities like every other kid and "Strep Throat" every year like clockwork. Early on I had tiny "tubes" put into my ears to help with drainage and alleviate my bouts of congestion. My tonsils and adenoids were also removed around this time. But, there were other kids in my grade who had the same procedures done. Totally normal right? Fast forward to age 15. I am an Honors Student and now a competitive dancer, rehearsing for 5 hours a day 4 days a week. Around this time, I started becoming very tired, even exhausted. I just blamed it on the school papers and crazy rehearsal schedule. I started gaining weight. I blamed this one on my hormones. I noticed more of my hair was falling out. Just a little more here and there not quite yet noticeable.

One day my mom noticed a bump, which looked like the size of a gum ball, in the middle to right side of my throat. Doctors and an ultrasound concluded that I had a goiter in my thyroid and several cysts in and around that area of my neck. The doctors, worried it was cancer, recommended that my entire thyroid be removed and that I be put on hormone replacement drugs for the rest of my life! I kindly thanked them for their advice but knew with my body at this age there had to be another way. We found a Naturopathic doctor and soon began changing my diet along with incorporating herbs. Not long after the goiter was not the visible bump it used to be, in fact there is not a bump at all. I had more energy and what seemed like a fog had lifted. As they say, "the rest is history". Since then I have been buried in books and research trying to further understand the connection between food and the body. It fascinates me, it is my passion, and it saved my life.

My intention for this book is to teach and show you simple choices you can make based on the key essentials throughout this book that will become the foundation for your health. I will show you how you can easily implement them in your daily life. You will notice more energy, clearer skin, looser fitting clothes and quicker recovery on the off chance you do get sick. My philosophy is: How can I become a better version of myself? And by "myself" I mean what is ideal for my body, in my life, with my career, family and schedule.

How to read this book

I would like to recommend that you read this book in order from cover to cover. It doesn't matter if you apply an essential a day or week at a time or jump in completely and start incorporating all at the same time. I have my 5 Day Jumpstart featured in this book to help solidify the choice you made for becoming healthier! Whichever you choose I still recommend reading the chapters in order because it is important to learn about these essentials first and how you can take steps to incorporate them second. With all that being said, I do encourage you to jump ahead to the recipe section and start cooking up some good food while you learn about your amazing body and what you can feed it for optimal health.

Section 1: Why you are feeling just ok and not optimal;

The Good, The Bad and The Just Plain Ugly

Chapter 1: The Good

We have all heard the term "You are what you eat" ... right? I am here to tell you it is 100% true! Simply put. The food or non-food substance we eat gets broken down by our teeth and if it's a carbohydrate, by our salvia, then it is further broken down by our stomach acid into little compounds and molecules. This makes it easier for our small intestine to do its job of grabbing the food particles and absorbing them into our blood stream. Once they are in our blood stream, they are taken to where they need to go in the body to use for energy, recovery, repair or storage. The particles of the food that do not get absorbed by the small intestine continue onto the large intestine where little bacteria "bugs" further dissolve the food to release nutrients for absorption. The large intestine also absorbs the water from the food and the rest is sent further south for excretion. Isn't this one of the coolest processes ever? The best part is, we do not even have to consciously tell our digestive tract and organs to do this. Our body takes care of us and has our best interests at heart. This is good news because we can alter our body just by the food we eat and even optimize this process by the quality of food we eat.

The other good news is that we live in a time and place where food availability has never been before. We do not have to hunt and gather every morsel of food we and our family eats. We also have access to clean water and it is pretty much instant access. We have years of experience and past generations help in teaching these processes to make it even better. We are beginning to understand and incorporate better practices in making food safer and delivering a variety of it to this melting pot of a country. There is also more and more farmers and shops labeling and suppling foods for challenged guts and/or health nerds, like me. Whether they are processed or natural, I can easily find a gluten free grain to cook spaghetti with or use a nut/seed substitute for dairy in a recipe. (We will go over the more natural and whole options for substitutions later in this book.) In a nut shell we have more access to food and a variety of food than any generation before us.

Chapter 2: The Bad

Now there are foods that mean well but behave most often badly for most people. I am talking about gluten, yeast, dairy, soy (unfermented), corn, caffeine, nuts and animal products just to name a few. These foods can be tolerated by some and can cause havoc for others. Even so, that these individuals become severally allergic to them. If you are someone who is severally allergic to anyone of these foods, you most likely already know; you experience sniffles, tongue swelling, hives or anaphylaxis immediately after eating the food. But what about if you are just mildly intolerant to them. Enough that you notice a sluggish feeling, upset tummy; gas or bloating, constipation or diarrhea, brain fog, troubled skin, headaches, joint and/or muscle pain. Most of this is caused by inflammation. Yes, food can cause inflammation. One of the ways this happens is when partially digested or broken down food (amino acid sequences), microbes, and/or toxins enter the blood stream through a compromised lining in the intestines. This can trigger the immune system to release inflammatory molecules and antibodies IgE, IgG, IgA, that act like bullets when defending the body. This process of course is meant to save us but if this process continues due to a malfunction and/or the over consumption of that substance, tissue can be damaged and many of the above symptoms can arise.

If you think you have a food sensitivity, I and many doctors recommend going on an elimination diet. You can do this carefully on your own but I always suggest talking it over with your doctor. Susan Blum, MD, MPH recommends a diet that eliminates the top 5 "bad" foods; gluten, dairy, soy, corn, and eggs for 3 weeks. Then reintroduce 1 at a time every 4 days to see if there is any reaction. She suggests that when you reintroduce the food to eat it several times a day for 2-3 days and observe. If you have a reaction right away, there is no need to continue eating it. To further heal your gut, I recommend restoring healthy intestinal flora to support digestion and removing the problem foods for at least 6 months, usually longer because immune cells have quite the memory. We will go over restoring a healthy gut in Section #2 Essential #3 Eat Whole Food.

The other factor that contributes to foods being "bad" is a concept called Bio-Individuality. This term was created by Joshua Rosenthal, MScED, and founder of Institute for Integrative Nutrition. "Diet should be based on the individual, not the theory". Bio-Individuality is a concept that one person's food is another person's poison. It is based on age, gender, race, ancestry, blood type, and level of activity. We learned a perfect example of this with food sensitivities. But let's take a closer look. All factors play into this theory but for this book I want to spend more time on blood type and ancestry. Those two factors I have found more success in helping myself and clients enable their body to heal itself. In the introduction to this book I explain my history with thyroid trouble! The Naturopathic Doctor that equipped me to heal myself first recommended eating foods aligned with what my blood type could tolerate. At the time I had no idea blood type even played a role but soon learned it made a huge impact on my health!

Here is a simple list of foods to reduce and increase based on your blood type. This is a simple guide adapted from the Institute for Integrative Nutrition. If this further interests you, I highly recommend reading "Eat Right for Your Type" by Dr. Peter J. D'Adamo yourself.

Type A:

Reduce: Meat, Dairy, Kidney beans, Lima beans, and Wheat

13

Increase: Vegetable Oil, Soy foods (preferably fermented), Vegetables, Seafood, Legumes, Fruit, Pineapple

Type B:

Reduce: Corn, Lentils, Peanuts, Buckwheat, and Wheat

Increase: Red meat (venison), Greens, Eggs, Liver, Vegetables, Legumes, and Fruit

Type AB:

Reduce: Red Meat, Kidney beans, Lima beans, Seeds, Corn, Buckwheat

Increase: Tofu, Seafood, Good quality dairy, Greens, Kelp, Fruit, Pineapple, Legumes, Vegetables

Type O:

Reduce: Wheat/Corn, Kidney beans, Lentils, Brussels sprouts, Cauliflower, Mustard

Increase: Kelp, Seafood, Salt, Liver, Red meat, Kale, Spinach, Broccoli, Pineapple

All foods are not created equal. Some can strengthen yet weaken others. It is important to look at all factors that make you, you. Along with blood type, ancestry is a crucial factor in figuring out which foods work for you and can help deconstruct your cravings. The parts of the world you are from and currently live in offer the best food to nourish your body. Think of the climate and environment you live in. Are you land locked and close to mountains or are you somewhere tropical either close to the ocean or fresh water? Also what you ate as a child can influence your cravings as an adult, think of comfort food.

Take some time out this week and observe your body's reaction to the food you eat. Are you sensitive to anything? Why could that be? I encourage you to stay in this zone of awareness as we go through this book.

Chapter 3: The Just Plain Ugly

The "Just Plain Ugly" List includes foods that should be avoided at all costs, or severely reduced! I am talking about the foods that are not food anymore. They have been processed, stripped and bleached of all nutrients and then sometimes, if we are lucky, have some or part of nutrients "enriched" – added back to them. I am all about cutting corners with preparation time and easy on the go foods but too much of these so called "foods" can wreak havoc on your endocrine, reproductive, digestive, nervous, and circulatory systems just to name a few. The reason being, if they have synthetic particles or only half the naturally occurring particles, our bodies cannot recognize it and therefore treat it as a threat. Sometimes this means getting rid of it ASAP or storing it in fat cells to protect the other cells and tissues. Have you ever heard of people talking about the "detox symptoms" are just as bad as "flu-like symptoms?" This is why! As we lose fat and "detox" our body we are releasing all of these toxins back into our systems and blood supply to then hopefully get rid of. The storage of these synthetic particles or toxins is also one of the many causes of cellulite. So many toxins are stuffed into fat cells that the cells begin to grow larger and be pushed to the outer layers of our skin creating a "bumpy" look and feel. These foods can be highly addictive and are hidden in a lot of well-known and used products.

The "Just Plain Ugly" List

- Refined sugar and/or High Fructose Corn Syrup (HFCS) and/or artificial sweeteners
- White flour and some canned goods
- Refined or hydrogenated vegetable oils
- Preservatives
- Additives such as Monosodium Glutamate (MSG), Butylated Hydroxyanisole (BHA), Butylated Hydroxytoluene (BHT)
- Artificial colorings and flavors
- "low" or "free" labeled foods: low-fat, fat free, sugar–free, decaf, even gluten free. I like to recommend grains that are naturally gluten free. (See Essential 3 in Section #2 for a list of naturally Gluten Free grains)
- Caffeine (Yes, I still love my cup of coffee but moderation and quality is key)
- Pesticides
- Genetically Modified Organisms (GMOS)

Please read food labels even on the packaged foods that are labeled "natural" or "healthy". There is little to no regulations on these words and they can be freely used on packaging and in marketing.

I also want to add Sugar! I know I briefly brought it up in the list above but I really want this food/ingredient to stand out on its own. We as humans are eating more sugar than ever before! Processed or non-processed sugar can take a toll on our liver and other organs! In Jason Wachob's article titled "Sugar can make you Dumb", he quotes this about sugar. "Studies conducted in 2012 concluded that eating too much sugar may also disrupt one's ability to think clearly due to impaired brain cell signaling." Jason Wachob, Mind Body Green Founder and CEO. Just think of the impact this has to your brain overtime. Sugar is also highly addictive! It is hidden in many foods especially the amounts. Sugar is not just in soda and candy anymore, it is in condiments, processed cereal, your favorite latte, canned foods and many of the foods in "fast food" chains contain sugar. I again plea with you to read your labels and look up how much exactly is a gram of sugar. When you see it with you own eyes it is unbelievable.

Section 2: The Key Essentials that can Change Your Life.

When I was diagnosed with a thyroid disorder and sought out a more natural approach in healing, one of the first things my doctor had me tackle was my diet. I incorporated a whole foods approach, meaning as little processed as possible as well as using my blood type as a guide. I cut out diary, gluten, many processed foods and ingredients. I also upped my vegetable intake and started cooking with and eating healthier fats. Once my system began getting stronger I started taking supplements and powerful herbs. I recommend getting a doctor's recommendation for supplements. They can be powerful healers but also everyone is different and having a doctor supervise is the best way to utilize them. Again these were supplements, they were a supplement to my already healthy diet change. This change did not happen overnight. Yes, I was sick and needed a change badly but I still had cravings for bagels and macaroni & cheese. What helped me the most was creating daily habits. I would focus on what I needed to feed my body that day and get into a habit of getting full on the good food so I didn't have to focus on the food that I had to cut out. This of course lead to other habits that helped me overcome my thyroid disorder.

This next section of the book is about my Top Five Essentials to a Healthy Life. These are the essentials that are building blocks for a healthy lifestyle. Making these essentials into habits will take determination and focus, but I promise it will be well worth it and this section is filled with support and tips to make the transition easy and delicious. These essentials are based on nixing inflammation (many cause for disorder and cravings in the body) and getting back to our roots. My approach is based on a holistic and traditional diet. (If you want to call it a diet) These 5 Essentials can easily be personalized and get you into a better and healthier body. Essential #1 we will look at Water! Easy right? I will go over the health benefits of good hydration and the side effects of dehydration. Plus delicious ways to drink more water. Essential #2 is all about Eating Whole Foods. We will go over five basic food groups and how to incorporate them into your diet. Essential #3 is going to be about Movement. We will discuss why movement is key for a healthy body and how to add more movement into your day. Essential #4 is one of my favorites and it is Self-Care. I will lay out what self-care is and why it is so important. Essential #5 is going to be fun because we will talk about how super foods can lead to Super powers. Ok not really, but they will help you feel more vitality and can help you recover from sickness and/or injuries quicker.

Also, for this section I have listed the Top 5 Essentials in order so they can easily become habits and build on one another. With that being said if one jumps out to you, please feel free to read about that one first. This is your book and your way of developing habits can differ from another.

Essential 1: Water

First and foremost, let's address our water intake. I will admit some days I rock this and some days I fall short. Part of the process of developing habits right? But what's the big deal with water? Why do we have to drink it and what exactly does it do for us? Water generates life, all life on earth. The human body is said to be composed of 25% solid matter and 75% water. The human brain is roughly 85% water. When we are dehydrated our cells act differently and may be the cause of body aches including backaches and headaches. Also many digestive problems may be linked to dehydration. Caffeine and alcohol are the biggest dehydrating agents. The amount of water recommended varies based on lifestyle factors such as age, weight, activity, climate, diet and health concerns. The USDA suggests to "let your thirst be your guide". I agree but also like to give my clients a starting point of drinking half your body weight in ounces of water a day. Start out with this as your goal and see how close you come to it and how you feel drinking that amount water. You can always decrease or increase this amount based on your lifestyle. Some factors that I suggest require more water is your activity level (during exercise), illness or infection, hot and/or humid climates, high altitude, if you are pregnant or breast feeding and if you have increased your alcohol and/or caffeine consumption. It is hard to notice if you are drinking too much water. If you are concerned I recommend speaking with your doctor on how much is required for you and your lifestyle.

I get that you might need to jazz up your water to make things a little more interesting. I love adding fruit and herbs to my water. They will infuse the water with their flavor and taste delicious all day. I recommend starting your day out with a cup of warm water with a squeeze of lemon and optional toss in of grated turmeric and/or ginger root. The raw natural powder version of those roots are fine too. Not only does this check off a cup of your water intake that day but it also is cleansing to the digestive tract. You can also count herbal tea into you water intake. Be mindful of the caffeine content, if it even does contain caffeine. Another great option is to add Certified Pure Therapeutic Grade essential oils to your water. Please be mindful of the quality of your essential oils. Some rank as low as perfume grade while others have many medicinal properties. More on Essential Oils in Section #2 Essential #5. Check the recipe section for more tips on jazzing up your water.

Essential 2: Eat Whole Food

Are you sitting down? Maybe with a glass of your deliciously fruit infused water next to you? If not, I encourage you too. This chapter is the most nutrient dense (pun intended) chapter of the book. It is packed full of easy tips and tricks to get you eating more whole foods with some science backing up why I recommend them. Are you ready?

Food, delicious and glorious food. It's almost a sin how much I love food and talking about food. The aroma of cooking, the laughter at the dinner table, and the gratitude towards God, the people and methods that it took to get this food to my plate. How can you not agree that food can feed us physically and emotionally? Yes, this chapter is more about the physical relationship we have with food but keep in mind when deconstructing cravings and creating your lifestyle that emotion and the longtime beliefs we have with food play a huge factor into your success with health. Without further ado, let's get into the Five Basic Food Groups I base my plans on to equip the body to change and heal.

These food groups are in no particular order; each person needs more of one than the other. Be mindful when incorporating these foods into your daily life and observe how you feel.

Plants

First up: plants. I like to categorize plants into 3 groups; leaves, ground and roots. Each have their own purpose and extraordinary line up of nutrients. Leaves, especially the dark green ones are vital to our health. They help give us sustained energy along with improving our circulation, respiratory and immune system. Dark leafy greens are even known to cleanse and improve liver, gall bladder and kidney function. Leafy greens can also help clear the paths of your excretory systems (skin, lungs, liver, colon & kidneys). Want beautiful, clear, smooth skin, up your greens intake. "Greens are the best source of alkaline minerals such as calcium, magnesium, iron, potassium, phosphorous, zinc, and vitamins A, C, E and K. They are loaded with fiber, folic acid, chlorophyll and many other micronutrients and phytochemicals." (Institute for Integrative Nutrition) All of those nutrients are abundant in whole leafy green vegetables. Eating as close as you can to organic and whole is best because it insures most of the nutrients are there and they can be easily absorbed by our digestive systems. Although organic is recommend in all food categories (insures safe growing and processing methods), eating non-organic greens and vegetables is better than eating none at all. Experiment with your green intake, if you get bored or feel overwhelmed start with a few of these; kale, collards, green and/or red leaf lettuce, spinach, Swiss chard, arugula, bok choy, cabbage, mustard greens, dandelion greens and herbs. (More on herbs in Essential #5) Keep in mind to rotate your greens to achieve better results and never feeling bored. Greens in their raw form supplies a refreshing number of live enzymes to your gut. Boiling or sautéing in water or oil helps the greens to "relax" so they are not as fibrous or pungent in flavor. I love to sauté kale, spinach or bok choy. Steaming greens can have the opposite effect. It can make the greens tight and allow to keep their fibrous texture. I recommend steaming bok choy and cabbage. Massaging greens with a homemade vinaigrette or simply lemon juice can help break down the fibrous texture and pungent flavor. My favorite is using lemon juice with kale for the base of my raw salads.

Some ground vegetables include zucchini, squash, pumpkin, broccoli, cauliflower, legumes, corn, rhubarb, Brussels sprouts, celery, cucumber, mushrooms, asparagus and many others. Many of these vegetables nourish our gut and bodies along with creating a balance between essential nutrients we need daily. Root vegetables include beets, ginger, turmeric root, carrots, turnips, parsnips, daikon, garlic, onions, potatoes and yams. I like to think of ground and root vegetables assisting us in obtaining hearty energy that also helps to "ground" us. Many of the vegetables in both categories like onions, yams, pumpkin, corn, beets and carrots are on the sweeter side. These sweet vegetables can help give the body lasting energy as well as fight off sugar cravings. You can chop, spiralizer, peel, dice, mince these vegetables to eat raw or sauté, steam, and bake to delicious goodness. My favorite way to prepare these types of vegetables is to bake at the least two of them with a protein. All that flavor with the addition of herbs in one baking sheet. Talk about efficient.

Proteins

The next food group is proteins. Proteins are made up of amino acids which are the building blocks for the majority of our human body. The consistent regulation and maintenance of the body is fueled by amino acids. Our bodies make some amino acids on its own and relies on food for the others. The amount and type of protein each individual needs are well, individual. Too little protein can lead to sugar cravings, fatigue, feeling weak and even spacey, as well as loosing healthy color and texture in hair and skin. Severe cases include inflammation and digestive disorders. Please contact a doctor if you think you are protein deficient. On the other hand too much protein can lead to dehydration, constipation, sugar cravings and huge imbalance of minerals and acidity in the body. This can put more pressure on digestive and elimination organs for filtration.

When deciding what type of protein to eat, keep in mind that it is highly personal. Some have emotional ties to not eating animal protein and some have cultural or ancestral ties to eating animal protein. Both animal and plant protein can benefit the human body, I personally choose to balance my intake of both. If you want to strictly get your protein and nutrition from plants I recommend eating a combination of plants including grains, seeds, nuts and vegetables to make sure your body is getting adequate amounts and variety of amino acids.

The basic types of protein include: animal meat like poultry, beef, lamb, bison, venison, mutton, and fish. Others include eggs, dairy and bee products. Some of the plant based protein options are whole grains, beans, soy, nuts, seeds, and even leafy greens. Like with your vegetable intake please change up what type of protein you are consuming. This will help insure that you are getting quality amounts of the different amino acids.

A word of caution about soy and dairy products. Soy products in America have been steadily gaining popularity. Even though soybeans are one of the most difficult beans to digest and many people are allergic to them. Soybeans are also one of the most genetically modified/engineered crop. When eating soy please keep it to the more natural, whole and organic form. Dairy, mostly cow's milk, is acid and mucus forming for many people. A lot of us have compromised digestive systems to where we lack the enzyme to break it down. I recommend eating different forms of dairy like yogurt (the cultures can help in digesting), butter, ghee (clarified butter, easier to digest) and even trying milk from goats and sheep. Dairy is an area I highly recommend buying organic due to the amount of growth hormones and antibiotics used in unnecessary means.

Fats

Now onto one of my favorite food groups...the fabulous fats. I say that because I want everyone to know that you can have a lean and healthy body when eating the right type and amount of fat. Healthy fats that have the right ratios of omega 3, 6 and 9 can fuel the brain as well as the body. Eating a diet that includes good fats like monounsaturated and polyunsaturated helps with organ function, energy, and beautiful skin. Monounsaturated fats are generally recommended to be eaten daily to help improve cholesterol. Some forms of monounsaturated fats include olive oil, nuts & seeds as well as halibut fish. Polyunsaturated fats are considered healthy and can be eaten often. They include flax seed/oil, walnuts, tuna, salmon and sardines. Polyunsaturated fats can also improve heart health and are considered anti- inflammatory. Saturated fats are healthy in smaller amounts. Some good saturated fats include beef, poultry, pork, dairy, coconut and avocados. Trans. fats should be avoided entirely. Some Trans. fats are in your processed foods such as margarine, candy, chips and baked goods. Please note that there are healthy substitutes we can make to help you transition away from trans-fat goodies.

Grains

Whole grains, key word whole have been around since early civilization. "They are an excellent source of nutrition, as they contain essential enzymes, iron, dietary fiber, vitamin E, and B-complex vitamins." (Institute for Integrative Nutrition) They are well known for providing long lasting energy. Quinoa is among my favorites due to its amino acid profile and long history of use. Some grains contain a protein called gluten. Gluten means "glue" in Latin, which is fitting because it is a binding agent in many breads, pastas and desserts. Gluten is the combo of two types of proteins called "gliadin and glutenin". It is mostly found in wheat, barley and rye. An increasing number of people are finding out they are gluten intolerant or even severely allergic to it. Some of the symptoms range from headache to upset stomach with diarrhea and in some severe cases vomiting. Medical professionals discovered this may be due to an autoimmune condition known as Celiac Disease. This happens when the consumption of gluten begins to deteriorate of the villi within the small intestine. Villi are small hair like tentacles that absorb nutrients from the food particles into our bodies. Not being able to absorb the nutrients from the foods we eat can lead to a bucket load of problems. This again is for the severe cases. For people who just experience a minor sensitivity to gluten, like myself, can experience gas/bloating, headaches and potential weight fluctuations. Even if you are not sensitive to gluten I recommend adding in some grains that are naturally gluten free like quinoa, brown/wild rice, amaranth, cornmeal/polenta, millet, buckwheat and oats. Oats and other naturally gluten free grains may be grown or processed in areas that grains with gluten are, and may become contaminated. It's best to do your research and read the label to double check. Grains are easy to prepare and easy to feed a whole family or have left overs. Usually 1 cup of dry grain yields 2-4 servings. For better digestion I recommend soaking them for 1-8 hours before cooking. Cooking grains consists of 1 cup grain to 2-3 cups water/broth or milk of choice, bringing it to a boil and letting it simmer. I love adding in herbs, spices and sea salt at this stage. Each grain has different cooking times; you can normally tell the grain is done when it looks like it has "popped" open or is easy to chew. Please read instructions carefully when buying your grains.

Cultured and Fermented Foods

I know I said "Fats" were my favorite food group but I love cultured and fermented food just as much. Especially after learning that they play a key role in gut health and the healing of a compromised one. Cultured foods are foods that contain or have live cultures added to them. Some of these live cultures are lactobacillus, bifidobacterium and saccharomyces boulardii. Our gut also contains these live cultures and is collectively known as the microflora or microbiome. Crazy spelled words that do crazy amounts of good for your gut. Yogurt and kefir are examples of cultured foods. Popular fermented foods are kimchi, pickles, and sauerkraut which also contain gut healthy bacteria. This is also where we get probiotics from. Probiotics are strains in certain foods that contain an adequate dose of live microbes. Probiotics also help in detoxing metals and toxins from the body. Prebiotics are foods that can resist the digestive acid in our stomach to make it to our intestine where they are fermented by intestinal microflora/bacteria. They then can actively restore gut balance and overall health with many digestive disorders. Probiotic rich foods include yogurt/kefir, miso (fermented soy), tempeh (fermented soy), sauerkraut, kimchi, pickles, beer, wine, olives, kombucha, buttermilk, raw vinegars and fermented meat and vegetables. Prebiotic rich foods include: onions, garlic, leeks, bananas, soybeans, asparagus, chives, peas, legumes, eggplant, honey, green tea, yogurt, cottage cheese and kefir. This list is adapted from Liz Lipski, PhD, CCN, CNS, LND. I always recommend getting your nutrients from whole foods but if you want to supplement with probiotics you totally can. Basic Probiotic supplements will have lactobacillus, streptococcus, and Bifidobacterium. All supplements have different dosages and mixes of the strains so please do your research on the product and the company before buying.

There we have it. Five Basic Food Groups to get you and your health back on track. Feel free to review them again and add a new food or ingredient to your grocery list each week. Like always be mindful of what you like and what your body leans towards. The perfect diet is a balance of each food group that fits your perfect body. Keep a food journal to track how you feel 30 minutes, 1 hour and 2 hours after eating a certain food or meal. You may want to try an elimination diet to further understand and potentially heal your system.

A few habits along with trying new foods each week would be to start buying local produce and products. It is not only better for your body but also your community. It connects us more to the area we live in and to the season we are in. Our bodies naturally crave heavier foods in the winter and lighter foods in the summer. Where ever you live bend these food groups to fit your location and climate. One more habit to start is meal prepping. It's not only for busy or body building people anymore. Meal prepping is cost effective and time efficient. It will also help keep you on track throughout the week AND weekend. You can start out simply by portioning out snacks such as nut/seed mixes for on the go as well as prepping some homemade hummus and chopped vegetables. I like to bake or grill some meats to easily add to my eggs in the morning or salads at lunch time. I also take the time to chop up vegetables and even roast some to quickly add to any dinners that week. You can boil a huge pot of grains that can be eaten throughout the week as breakfast or as a side dish. I also love fermenting my own vegetables. Taking a Sunday to prep them and just watch and maintain them all week can yield bucket loads of fermented vegetable goodness for weeks to come. Check out the recipes in the back of the book and see which ones you can increase to make enough for 2-3 days after. Try to eat raw chopped vegetables and fruit quicker. Once they are cut or juiced they will oxidize and slowly lose nutritional value. Take some time adding and planning out these new habits into your lifestyle. Go at your own pace and remember even small steps are steps forward.

Essential 3: Movement

Let's first bust the myth of calories in vs calories out! Take an apple, 1 medium red apple is almost 100 calories. Now compare that to 100 calorie processed snack pack. Which one will most likely give you more nutrients and energy for the same calories? Also the red apple will be digested and absorbed fully. We already know that some of the chemicals in the processed snack pack might not be able to be digested and absorb but rather stored. Now let's factor in movement. People who sit at a desk for 8+ hours a day will and should eat different than a nurse or waitress that is on their feet all day. Also take into consideration your workout routine. Does it exist at all or are you a professional athlete? Do you prefer long distance training or something like High Intensity Interval Training? Different movement has different effects on our body and how we store energy (food we eat). Keep in mind that different movement effects different people.

Through my training at the Institute for Integrative Nutrition and outside research, I have found all movement can be beneficial at different times. Say you are feeling tight, stressed and are experiencing a "hot" demeanor. I would recommend that you to take a walk or yoga/Pilates class. Your body is crying out for rest and restorative movement. Take the time to stretch and bend the body while being mindful and in a calm state. Now say you are feeling expansive, sluggish, and scatter brained. You might need a quicker paced and higher intensity workout to help balance you. By nature, I am the latter most of the time; expansive and scatter brained. Probably has something to do with my thyroid leaning toward the sluggish side, but that is my opinion based on observation. I set up my week knowing that I am slothful on Monday, tense by Thursday and energetic on the weekends. I plan my workouts around what my body and mind need.

Along with balancing my workouts around my energy I also choose workouts based on how I want to store energy, food. This has helped me to shed weight, increase lung and heart function as well as think clearer. A lot of what I talk about pertaining to exercise comes from studying Dr. Al Sears M.D. work and his P.A.C.E. Program. For better understanding lets break down the mechanisms in the body that are activated when you work out and how they help you after you work out.

Your body has the option to select energy from fat, carbohydrates like glycogen or by breaking down proteins. The amount of time and the intensity at which you work out tells the body where to get its energy from. In the beginning of your work out your body will use something called ATP (Adenosine Tri- Phosphate) which is the most readily available source of energy. After a few minutes your body switches to carbohydrates for the next 15-30 minutes before it switches to fat.

This is where most in the fitness industry would say cardio at moderate intensity, lasting more the 30-60 minutes is the most effective because you enter the fat zone meaning you are burning fat for fuel while exercising. Makes some sense but not to the body. Our bodies are designed to adapt for survival. If you are consistently getting the body in "fat burning zone" your body will adapt to storing the food you eat as its adapted main source of energy... fat.

"Our bodies actually burn more fat while resting and restoring the inner workings of our bodies, roughly 60% energy used in this case is from fat. We burn a higher percentage of carbs (which are readily stored in muscle tissue) while at low intensity exercise like walking or yoga/stretching." (McArdle W.D. 1999 Sports & Exercise Nutrition. NY Lippincott Williams & Wilkins) In other words, how you exercise stimulates an adaptive response in the body to store the kind of energy you need for the kind of activity you perform.

Let's take a closer look at why this is so important. When you are engaging in low intensity activity you are able to breathe in enough oxygen to continuously combine with carbs, fats and proteins to make ATP. So your body will always have enough readily available ATP to use for energy. When you are engaging in a higher intensity activity like sprinting your body will run out of ATP quicker due to the lack of sufficient oxygen to activate the processes in making ATP. This is also called anaerobic meaning without oxygen. This system can sustain you in a sprint but not for long. It is when you stop you will notice your heart is pumping and you are panting in order to get adequate amounts of oxygen to start replenishing ATPs. In doing this you are creating an adaptive response for your body to store food in a more readily available form.

Short bursts of intense exercise, will teach your body to burn energy stored in your muscles instead of fat because this type of energy is released quicker. This also means while you rest you will be burning more fat to prepare for the next workout. This is also called "after burn". The University of Missouri found that short bouts of exercise were more effective for lowering fat and triglyceride levels in the blood. High triglycerides dramatically increase your risk of heart disease. (Press Release. Short bouts of exercise reduce fat in bloodstream. American College of Sports Medicine. Aug 5 2004)

For quicker and better results, you can progressively change a factor in your short bursts of activity. For example, each burst you sprint faster and harder or up the incline/resistance. Like I said before when I set up my weekly workouts I take into account what my body needs (higher intensity work out or a more restorative workout) but I keep in mind these principles. I love to create circuits that bounce between high intensity movements and strengthening movements like for example squat jumps and walking lunges. You can also use these principles in creating a set of sprints either outside, on a treadmill, bicycle or even while swimming. Below are a few of my favorite circuits to do for my high intensity days. On low intensity days, I will take a walk or do some light yoga/Pilates/dance inspired movement.

*Please talk with your doctor to see if you are healthy enough for physical activity. Always know you can start much smaller and have longer recovery times or even just begin by doing 2-3 sets. It's all individual and you will become stronger.

Body Weight Circuits: 45 secs work, 15 secs rest or 12-15 reps, rest until your heart/breathing rate become normal.

Example: Squats, V-Crunches, Push-ups, plank. Do as many reps as you can of each in 45 secs and rest for 15 secs in between. You can do that whole set again 2-3 more times. You can switch up the exercises to include jumping jacks, jump squats, Russian twists and triceps dips.

Essential 4: Self Care

This chapter is all about focusing on the food that isn't on your plate. The ones that feed your soul! In this book I am not going to get super spiritual or as deep as a yoga retreat but there is something to be said about the act of self-care and how it can influence our health. At the Institute for Integrative Health I learned about "Primary Foods" and how they can fuel and feed us more completely than food. Think of a time you were in love. Life was exciting, you were glowing and food became secondary. Or a time when you were so focused and excited about a new project you just forgot to eat. Career, Relationships, Spirituality along with Physical Activity are examples of Primary Food. When these factors are out of balance, no amount of kale can completely heal you. When I advise my clients to practice self-care I first have them take a closer look at those four main categories. Maybe write down a few things they love about it and a few things they could change about It. Being able to observe and acknowledge that these areas in your life can impact your health can be the turning point for your healing.

Another act of self-care is simply the act of taking time for yourself. Take the time to prepare an amazing meal for yourself or loved one. Take the time to relax in a hot bath or get to bed early. Go get a massage, facial or read a book. Go take a dance class or have a pickup basketball game with your friends. Even just a few moments during the day that you can dedicate to yourself and meditate, pray or write a note of all the things you are grateful for is self-care. One un-seemingly monumental act of self-care is simply saying no. Saying no to things or situations that do not serve you. This is easier said than done but seriously. If you say yes to every project, opportunity, event or person that came your way you would not get anything accomplished. Take some time, know your priorities and for a season say no to all that will hinder you from success.

Every morning I take a few moments to pray and thank God for all that I am grateful for. I also like to envision myself accomplishing my goals and experience that excitement and gratitude. I then will pray for that same excitement and accomplishment to extend to my family and friends. That they too will be successful and happy. After this is done how can I not be happy and grateful?

One more act of self-care I love is called the "Hot Towel Scrub". This can be done anytime of the day. If you do it in the morning it will help to invigorate you, if you do it before bed it will also calm you. All you need is a sink or bowl of hot water and a wash cloth. You will submerge the cloth into the hot water and wring out. While the cloth is still hot and steamy you will begin to scrub the skin gently. Do one section of the body at a time, beginning with fingers and hands. Working your way up both arms to your shoulders, neck face and chest. Continue on your upper back, abdomen, and so on until you reach your toes. All the while continuing to dip the cloth in the hot water to keep it hot and steamy.

The "Hot Towel Scrub" creates a profound and loving relationship with the body even the parts we have trouble accepting. This act also helps to open pores to release toxins, promotes circulation and activates the lymphatic system both helping to reduce cellulite. It will also help to reduce muscle tension and can calm the mind. I love doing this before I go to bed, especially with a drop or two of Lavender Essential Oil in the water. A good night's sleep is guaranteed.

Self-care can be easy and effective on your journey towards health. Schedule one or two acts of self-care a week and go from there.

Essential 5: Superfoods, Super herbs & Essential Oils

The number of superfoods, herbs and essentials oils is vast and the research behind them is ever growing. Part of my protocol for a better supported thyroid was to incorporate a combo of superfoods, herbs and essential oils along with the lifestyle change I spoke of earlier. I still to this day incorporate all three to help continue my journey towards health and vitality. What I have found is beyond remarkable and I have my health to prove it. In this section I will go over my top favorites in each and explain how you can incorporate them into your day for optimal wellness and supercharged health.

"Superfoods are a class of the most potent, super-concentrated, and nutrient-rich foods on the plant. They are the optimum choice for improving overall health, boosting the immune system, elevating serotonin production, enhancing sexuality, cleansing, lowering inflammation and alkalizing the body." (David

Wolfe) For the simplicity of this book I am just going to give you my 5 favorite Superfoods. There is so much more than this and if you are interested in pursuing superfoods more I highly recommend David Wolfe's book "Super Foods". My top Five Superfoods are Cacao, Maca, Bee Products, Sea Vegetables/Micro-Algae and Goji Berries.

Cacao is the nut/seed of a fruit of an Amazonian tree which is the base for what we know and love as chocolate. I know, surprise, you can have chocolate. But not just any chocolate! Try to find ones that are close to the original form of cacao as possible. The closer you are the better for you it will be. Cacao is one the highest antioxidant foods on the plant. It boosts magnesium, iron, manganese and chromium. "Raw chocolate improves cardiovascular health, builds strong bones, is a natural aphrodisiac, elevates your mood and energy and increases longevity."*

Maca is generally sold as a fine powder made from the root of the plant that has been dried. There are many folk tales surrounding this superfood as being a part of the "coming of age ceremonies" for men in its native land, the Peruvian Andes. "Dried Maca powder contains more than 10% protein and nearly all 20 amino acids, including the seven essential amino acids."* This superfood has been known to increase endurance, energy, strength and libido. I love to add a good quality Maca powder to my smoothies. It blends well with raw cacao and makes for an energy boosting drink. Maca has a strong earthy flavor and is very potent in nutrients. If you are just starting out, please be cautious and start with only ¼ tsp and slowly increase from there. It is best to stop at 2 tbsp. but keep checking in with how you feel and always speak with you doctor or health care professional for further guidance.

Bee Products, mostly Bee Pollen has strengthened my health and given me noticeable energy. Bee Pollen is said to be the most complete food found in nature. Huge statement but get this, "bee pollen contains nearly all the B vitamins, especially B- 9 (folate) and all 21 essential amino acids, making it a complete protein."* Bee Pollen can be a lot to take in, flavor and potency wise. Just like Maca, I recommend you start small with your daily amount of bee pollen. I have added a teaspoon to smoothies and taken it in a capsule form. Honey is another bee product I cannot live without. It is not only used as a sweetener but seen by many as a superfood. In its raw and purist form (wild and unfiltered), honey is rich in minerals, antioxidants, probiotics and enzymes. Again, please listen to your body and speak with your doctor. Some people can handle sweeteners and some cannot.

Sea vegetables such as kelp, dulse, and nori are rich in trace minerals and nutrients that are both pulled from the ocean and sun. "Sea vegetables help remove heavy metals, detoxify the body of radioactive iodine, regulate immunity and decrease the risk of cancer."* Sea vegetables are especially excellent in supporting the endocrine system including the thyroid, adrenals and hormones as well as the immune system. Micro-Algae has gained popularity in the supplement world recently and for good reason. Spirulina and AFA Blue- Green Algae are vital superfoods. Surprisingly enough Spirulina is the highest source in the world of complete protein (65%). Not only that but it also contains minerals, phytonutrients and enzymes. "AFA blue- green algae is a wild-grown superfood that is made up of 15% blue pigmented phycocyanin which, according to Christian Drapeau in his book Primordial Food, increases our internal production of stem cells."*

Goji berries have been used in Traditional Chinese Medicine for over 5,000 years. These berries are known for their link to longevity and to strength building. This superfood contains 18 kinds of amino acids, including eight essential amino acids, 21 trace minerals, antioxidants, iron, polysaccharides and vitamins such as B and E. I have found good quality dried goji berries at the local health food store and love to add them to my morning porridge, salads, trail mix and use them as toppings on my smoothies.

According to *The Herb Society of America's New Encyclopedia of Herbs and Their* Uses by Deni Bown: a herb is a small, seed bearing plant with fleshy, rather than woody, parts. They are valued for their flavor, fragrance, medicinal and healthful qualities, economic and industrial uses, pesticide properties and coloring materials. Herbs and spices have been used for over thousands of years in treating and supporting the human body back to health. Just like superfoods they are packed with antioxidants, minerals and life-giving nutrients. I add herbs in my cooking, tea mixtures and take them as supplements. Turmeric, ginger, basil, dandelion, parsley, oregano, rosemary, thyme, black pepper, cayenne, cinnamon, mint, and Echinacea just to name a few. If you are new to using herbs, take it little by little and have fun experimenting with your food. If you are interested in taking them as dietary supplements please talk to your doctor, they are very potent and some are better when taken for a short period of time.

Essential Oils are in a class of their own. Yes, they are from some of the foods and herbs I listed above but more specifically they are volatile aromatic compounds that are found in seeds, leaves, stems, bark, roots, and flowers of a plant. They protect the plant against environmental threats and give off a beautiful fragrance. These valuable oils have been traded and used since before Jesus's time. Some were even worth more than gold. Essential Oils, when grown and distilled for purity, potency and efficacy are 50-70 times more potent than herbs. For example: 1 drop of peppermint essential oil is roughly equivalent to 28 cups of peppermint tea. They can be used in food preparation, beauty treatments, and personal perfume, house cleaning products, bug repellants, and can be beneficial to every system in the human body. Essential oils can be used aromatically, topically and internally. When essential oils are diffused or inhaled they can be very stimulating or calming to our system. They can open air ways, support our respiratory system and cleanse the air around us. Essential oils can also be used on the skin and massaged for therapeutic benefits. Their chemical structure enables them to pass through the skin almost immediately. Some essential oils can be added to your food to not only boost flavor but medicinal benefits as well. Some may even be used internally to support a healthy lifestyle and should be taken with extra caution. **

I use many different essential oils through-out the day countless times and for dozens of reasons. For the purpose of this book I will just share the ones that can boost your health and get you started. Peppermint, lemon, grapefruit and coriander among many

41

other things support the digestive tract. Cinnamon, grapefruit and clary sage help to support healthy hormone function. Clove, melaleuca, lavender, oregano, and most citrus oils work to support our immune system. **

*Institute for Integrative Nutrition Source

** These statements are not regulated by the FDA and are not intended to treat or cure any disease. I throw a word of caution out that not all essential oil companies are the same and their oils/products are nowhere near the same. Essential oils can be powerful and beautiful healing compounds but there is not a system or committee (like the F.D.A.) put into place to inspect and set standards for growers and producers of essential oils worldwide. From growing to harvesting to distilling and distributing many damaging things can happen to these amazing compounds and in turn may be harmful to you. Be sure to work with a company that only produces pure and safe essential oils. I have worked with essential oils for over 5 years and have tried dozens and researched many. To find out which company I trust and use please find me on Social Media at Whole Essentials. Please contact a doctor or health care professional on essential oils and herbs.

Section 3: 5 Day Jumpstart & Five Ingredient or Less Recipes

5 Day Jumpstart

Morning Tea: Cup of hot water with 2 minced/mashed peppermint leaves and juice from ½ squeezed lemon. May add grated roots of turmeric or ginger.

Evening Tea: Cup of hot water with 1 tsp organic cinnamon and juice from ¼ squeezed orange.

Day 1:

Breakfast: Smoothie

Snack: 1 piece of fruit or 1 cup of green tea

Lunch: Basic Kale Salad

Snack: Chia Seed Pudding

Dinner: Salmon Bake

Day 2:

Breakfast: Eggs over Hash

Snack: 1 piece of fruit or 1 cup of green tea

Lunch: left over Salmon Bake

Snack: Chia Seed Pudding

Dinner: Basic Kale Salad with added protein (grilled chicken or fish)

Day 3:

Breakfast: Brown Rice and Quinoa Porridge

Snack: 1 cup Berry Salad

Lunch: Quinoa Salad

Snack: 1 cup of Sauerkraut or Fermented Salad

Dinner: Sweet and Savory Chicken Dinner

Day 4:

Breakfast: left over Brown Rice and Quinoa Porridge

Snack: 1 cup Berry Salad

Lunch: 1 bowl of Butternut Squash Soup

Snack: 1 cup of Sauerkraut or Fermented Salad

Dinner: Sweet and Savory Chicken Dinner

Day 5:

Breakfast: Smoothie

Snack: 1 piece of fruit or 1 cup of green tea

Lunch: 1 Bowl of Butternut Squash Soup

Snack: 1 cup Berry Salad

Dinner: Ground Buffalo/ Turkey with Roasted Veggies

> *Due to seasons changing and preferences you can exchange snacks for berries, grapefruit, pear, apple, figs as well as having more chia seed pudding or fermented salad instead.

Five Ingredient or Less Recipes

Infused Water:

- In a quart sized jar add 1 lime sliced with fresh peppermint leaves
- In a quart sized jar add 1 grapefruit sliced with ¼ cup raspberries
- In a quart sized jar add ½ cup frozen mixed berries

Breakfast:

Smoothie

- 1 cup frozen blueberries
- 1- 2 tbsp. seeds (chia, flax, hemp)
- 1 cup Almond or Coconut milk (if using canned coconut milk only use ¼ cup milk with ¾ cup water)
- 1 cup dark leafy greens
- Optional 1 scoop of protein… my favorite is chocolate! (helps to hide flavor of greens)
- Add ingredients to a high speed blender and blend away!

Eggs over Hash

- 1-2 whole eggs
- ¼ cup each of 2-3 vegetables (mushrooms, onions, bell peppers, spinach, tomatoes etc)
- ½ cup boiled or roasted sweet potatoes
- Pinch or two of sea salt
- 1 tbsp. fresh basil (add when plating)

- Prep sweet potatoes the night before by either boiling them or roasting them until they are soft can add sea salt. Sauté desired vegetables to top the sweet potatoes. Cook eggs in grass fed butter, ghee, olive oil or coconut oil and add on top of vegetable mixture. Top with fresh basil.

Brown Rice and Quinoa Porridge

- ¼- ½ cup each of cooked brown rice and quinoa
- Grass fed butter or ghee
- Dash or two of cinnamon, vanilla or maple syrup
- ¼- ½ cup almond milk
- ¼ cup chopped soaked almonds
- Optional to add 1 scoop of protein
- Add all ingredients to heated grains, stir and enjoy.

Lunch:

Kale Salad (makes 2 servings)

- 2 cups Kale (usually 1 bunch)
- 1 beet spiralized or chopped
- ¼ chopped red onion
- 1 cup cooked quinoa
- 1 chopped bell pepper
- Dressing: juice from 1-2 lemons, 2 tbsp. olive oil, 1 tbsp. apple cider vinegar (can add 1-2 tbsp. of agave or maple syrup)

Quinoa Salad

- 1 cup cooked quinoa
- 1-2 cups chopped raw or sautéed vegetables (green or red onions, mushrooms, Brussel sprouts, broccoli, sweet potatoes, bell peppers, green beans and/ or asparagus
- Dashes of fresh basil or parsley
- Pinch of Sea Salt
- Optional add in of protein (Chicken, buffalo or beef)

Butternut Squash Soap (makes 3-4 servings)

- 1 medium yellow onion
- 2 tbsp. olive oil
- 4 garlic cloves
- 4 cups vegetable broth
- 1 medium to large Butternut Squash
- Sea salt and pepper to taste
- Optional add in of 1 tbsp. pumpkin spice seasoning
- sauté onions and garlic in big stew pot with olive oil. Add broth and squash. Bring to boil then let simmer until squash is soft. Blend and enjoy.

Dinner:

Salmon Bake

- Salmon filet
- Kale
- 1 lemon sliced, sea salt and pinch or two of fresh ginger
- Vegetable bed can be any 1-2 of these (asparagus, green beans, Brussel sprouts or broccoli)
- Paired with ¼- ½ cup cooked quinoa
  Layer vegetables under fish and top fish with ½ cup kale, 3 lemon slices and fresh ginger. Can add sea salt and 1-2 tbsp. grass fed butter, ghee or olive oil. Wrap in tin foil

and bake or grill until fish is flaky and vegetables are tender.

Sweet and Savory Chicken Dinner

- Baked chicken or turkey breasts (grass fed butter, ghee or olive oil)
- Boiled or roasted yams/ sweet potatoes or squash
- Plate hot and add fresh or dried tarragon leaves

Ground Meat and Roasted Vegetables

- ½- 1 cup Ground buffalo, beef or turkey cooked in grass fed butter, ghee or olive oil
- 2 cups roasted vegetables (broccoli, Brussel sprouts, carrots, mushroom, onions, sweet potatoes
- ¼- ½ cup cooked quinoa or brown rice
- Sea salt and black pepper
- Optional to add Fermented Salad as a side

Snacks and Desserts:

Berry Salad

- 3 cups mixed berries (strawberries, blue berries, black berries, raspberries)
- ¼ cup soaked almonds (soaked for 8 hours in water)
- ¼ cup soaked walnuts (soaked for 8 hours in water)
- Can add toppings like cinnamon, coconut shavings, honey or even coconut sugar
- Mix and enjoy

Chia Seed Pudding

- 1 cup almond or coconut milk
- 3 tbsp. chia seeds
- Can add toppings like cinnamon, coconut shavings, honey, banana, pumpkin puree, blended or fresh fruit and/ or 1 tbsp. cacao powder (chocolate)

Fermented Salad (makes about 4 servings)

- 4 cups vegetables (green or purple cabbage, beets, carrots, celery or cucumbers)
- 1 tbsp. and a pinch of sea salt
- Add sea salt as you chop desired vegetables, push mixture down into a quart sized mason jar, make sure there is little to no oxygen (can add vegetable mixture to top of jar) cover with a cloth secured by a rubber-band. Let sit for 1-3 weeks. The flavor will slightly change so feel free to taste as you go once a week has passed.

Spicy Mocha Night Cap

- 1 cup almond milk
- 1 tbsp. cacao powder (chocolate)
- 1 tsp. cinnamon
- 1 tbsp. maple syrup
- 1 tbsp. grass fed butter or ghee
- Heat almond milk, cacoa, cinnamon and maple syrup in a sauce pan. Add butter and blend. (blending will create froth and a better taste)
- Optional to add 1 tsp. maca powder and 2/3 cup coffee with 1/3 almond milk and have in the morning.

Thank you for reading this book. I hope it brought you healing and joy. Please connect with me on Social Media at Whole Essentials.

Author Biography

Tiffnee Wertenberger grew up in Small Town USA. Moving from Wyoming to Michigan then to Colorado, she has been surrounded by nature. Being diagnosed with a thyroid disorder early on in high school, she began her journey back to health. Tiffnee's love of dance took her to Los Angeles, California where she worked as a professional dancer on the set of many music videos and T.V. shows. All the while still forging her path to health. With her experience in the dance industry and the overcoming of a thyroid disorder, Tiffnee left Hollywood and searched for a way to share her story with the want to help others. Tiffnee has completed and earned a Certificate in Nutrition and Health Coaching from the Institute of Integrative Nutrition. Due to the amount that herbs had helped in the healing of her thyroid, she decided to study those plants and their essential oils to where she received a Certification in Basic Essential Oil History and Application from Franklin University. Tiffnee now lives in Colorado sharing what she has learned and working with individuals who are forging their own path to health.

www.ingramcontent.com/pod-product-compliance
Lightning Source LLC
Chambersburg PA
CBHW070226290526
45789CB00004B/1522